Dedication

This book is dedicated to me for surmounting my own struggles. It was like I was never going to find myself out of the maze porn addiction created in my life. A struggle of twenty years

was overcome in days. Glory

be to God almighty.

Porn and Love

The trial of a man doesn't begin suddenly. Like everyone, I was another hypocrite. The hard-worn balcony of our hostel has seen an assembly of men over the years. Day after day, students will sit around in the evening to discuss what the lost boys usually talk about.

"I will never do that, bruh! There are so many women"

he had said. We knew how farfetched those words were, but we took it to be a fact. I think in every circle of thieves, fact, no matter how false it might be, is the truth. Then, the conversation took a deeper assessment of the issue. My voice couldn't have been louder. And my interest couldn't have been more obvious. Other boys tried to show how much they destest the act. I felt we knew the truth much more than we could ever admit. The loudest drum probably needed tuning. We needed tuning. Our enemy is a universal one.

The truth that evades you lies in the little things. My first year at the university was beyond what I had imagined. You see, I had thought of a place where freedom gives more of everything especially social life. Yes, I was right. i was wrong. I came from a lower class of the social hierarchy. I was not equipped with the necessary resources to live the social life of my dream. So, like most people like me, I dreamt.

My school was a public school. It was an exceptionally designed higher institution for the poor. It was a place for the middle class too. Maybe I should think of my family as a middle-class one. The truth is the line between the poor and the middle class was and still is a thin one. Easily eroded and the mobility up and down these classes is rapid. There were super poor.

In my school, one or two times you will find children from rich homes. They were few but now and then they popped up. They tend not to be easily known because they were usually the black sheep of politicians. Yes! Politicians are stupendously rich.

Soon enough, when I got to the university I understood my economical state wasn't going to get the life I had been craving. I quickly realized I wasn't going to see an alternative either. The only option left for people like me was hoping to score based on the look. And perhaps, academic prowess. Did I possess any or the two of these? NO! How could I? I spent the bulk of my class time daydreaming about the social life I couldn't have. In my dreams, I wore the latest baggy and had my hair in dread. My shirts were mostly parsley and I drove a Camry car with tinted windows and drank bottled water.

It wasn't that others like me don't get to have fun. I did have fun. I had plenty of fun.

But the fun came in different ways for people like us. A man at ease in a position will soon find joy in the matching objects the position grants. But the life that matches our class, status a resource wasn't what we wanted. We looked beyond what we could afford. I didn't stop at what I could get, perhaps it was a human thing. I will forever seek what is beyond me.

My first time using porn was on a Saturday afternoon. I had dashed home from school skipping about three classes because I felt low on motivation. I met a lady a day earlier and every conversation and gesture pointed to mutual interest. It was like I had scored one out of my league. The night was restless as the thought of what my relationship with her was going to be like filled my heart. There was no room to think about what we were not going to be like. I thought about so many ways to make myself appealing. I thought I needed to give a strong signal; the primitive male instinct. What is now called zahavian signal? But in the end, I was going to make myself appealing in the best way I could. My clothing was different that day, and I had gotten to the class before anybody. I didn't know at that time that I was giving much more than I could ever realize.

The class became filled up. Students pandering here and there, discussing whatever they fancied. I had positioned myself near her usual spot and I knew no way she could have missed my presence. Few people gawked at me. I had sat there before and there is an explanation for that. I am one of the people that do wonder why some students tried so hard to be inconspicuous. The row I sat in was one of the ridiculously positioned rows in the classroom sitting positions. It was an arc form of rows, facing the teacher's pedestal. I gives an ample view of the class also while facing the door fully.

She came in and saw me and immediately the reality hit me. It was like I had not existed. She walked by exchanging pleasantries with fellow students all around me. She looked at me and said "hi". Like the one you give people you know but not known.

It was like there was an eruption in me that the fantasy I circled in my brain had held at bay. I felt like I need to take a breath, but it wasn't the air that I needed.

I was like an overstretched balloon begging for a pop. Everything became boring, I felt antsy and needed to relieve myself and sleep so I can circle back to a fresh me.

There was a reason I felt that way. Some of you must have reached that stage differently, but always end in one way: Porn and nut.

I took the first bus back home. Feeling justified for what I was about to go do. The anticipation was intense. I dashed into my room and in one swift movement slotted the hinge at the back of the door. Oh! No one can barge in now. I brought out my blackberry and off to work I went. It wasn't like I had not watched porn before, but I had not taken it functionally as I decided that day. It wasn't a light action, deep in ignorance. It was a gateway for me now, a primary stimulant to a secondary one; masturbation.

For over four hours indulge in porn of all kinds and wearily, I climaxed. For a few days, it was like a fix for me, my getaway drug from the emptiness I felt. Over the months I became dependent on it, going on and off. A slight misunderstanding could tilt me down the slippery hole of porn and masturbation.

While I searched for a partner, I continued in my habit. Somehow I felt like it relieved. It made having a partner not much of a big deal to me. I haven't fixated on a physical partner like that again.

Why Porn is Dangerous

Ever hear the advice to "never trust easy"? In essence, Easy disobeys the sowing and reaping principle. You are intended to pay a price for the effort you put in and receive in return. Porn is dangerous primarily due to how widely accessible it is and how intense it is. All of them together with the fact that masturbation is a combined act. For me, watching porn was the simplest way to get sexy. I always reached for my Blackberry whenever I felt lonely. My browsing history was ugly. You'll read captions like, "Teenage girl gangbanging next door when her mother was home," a married black kid from Brazil who is freed by him" Caught a Hostel Neighbor Fingering and Fucked in Ass." Disgusting captions that reek of degradation. Whatever is worth having in life will not come easy. My friend porn is easy. Porn is easy in its entirety; from getting it to using it. I could say the bigger part of my life in college was lost because I watched porn a lot and masturbated often. The problem was I didn't know how much it was hurting me. The clarity that comes after I have ejaculated to a bout of porn wasn't usually long-lasting. It is a euphoria of pleasure because it's never long-lasting. I thought it helped me concentrate. It in fact made me dependent on it to feel good and deprived me of a much healthy way of concentrating.

I soon realized that I had lost interest in some porn scenes and crave scenes more extreme. I spent a considerable length of time looking for that particular scene. The one that gives me a jolt of pleasure. Trust me I would have covered so many before I get close to anyone to make me feel good. Whenever I did get close to one, the scene becomes my go-to for the time being. It could be a porn channel about school teens (by the way that's a very popular tag in the porn world). Sometimes scenes of older grandma, anal amateur, etc. I will quickly develop a relationship with these channels that when have surfed for porn for hours I will come back to them to cap it up and get off. They become the easing valve. But only for the time being. I will soon outgrow these and by that time I had already gotten hooked on other extreme ones.

It took me years to understand what I had been doing to my brain and body. With each porn I used and with each act of masturbation, I reprogrammed myself. I wired my brain to look for the easy way out in the easy-to-get gratification. The scientific explanation for this is dopamine dynamics. Neuroscientists positioned that dopamine is the molecule responsible for drive, desire, and craving. It is a molecule responsible for carrying out or doing stuff that your brain thinks will in the end be rewarding. This is how the human brain recognizes activities that are good or bad. Or pleasing and uninteresting. If an action is interpreted as rewarding for survival, there is a release of dopamine. this in turn releases the sensation of pleasure.

It's basically a feel-good molecule that tells the brain the kind of pleasure the body is experiencing. The problem is; dopamine is a noninfinite yet renewable resource. A pool that can be significantly reduced but renewable. But, there is a threshold for dopamine and it can be depleted beyond the threshold. It can go far up and crash down below a baseline. Activities like porn consumption will significantly trigger dopamine. Since it's a mirror-symmetrical process (the higher it goes, the lower it comes), it crashes below the baseline afterward. This will result in deeps in afterward activities. Porn will juggle you between peak and crash and this can be instrumental to depression.

With the pleasure of dopamine and the

availability of porn, the brain moves you to indulge in it more by searching for more arousing porn to give you a dopamine hit. A level of tolerance is developed to past experiences, so you search for more novel porn. Novelty itself is a sexual kick.

The intricate apparatus that is the brain is intended to process everything in moderation. The nerves that makeup it are primarily those that are organically intended to keep us alive and protected. We should be aware that our bodies' natural instinct is to seek out ways to survive, and they will always tend in that direction. This contributes to porn consumption since the brain sometimes confuses survival with wants. The problem is that the brain only has a limited capacity for dopamine. It loses sensitivity when given a dose that is higher than usual. By doing this it has taken in the right amount of dopamine. Since what gives it the right amount of dopamine doesn't give it again, the only way we know is to up our game. Then we consume more porn and masturbate the more thereby bombarding the brain with more dopamine. Eventually it get tired of that too and need more to make us feel good. That's the basis of addiction essentially. It is a urge that keeps asking for more.

When I became exposed to porn I was 19 years old. That was then. The internet started becoming a thing in my country. That was around 2007. It has been revealed that children as young as 11 now have free access to porn. This implies that by 13 these children have already created caches of porn videos and digital relationship that is harmful to them. Porn is at our fingertips now. It is in everything you see. Porn availability at this time is so prevalent. Andrew Ferebee said that we are the first generation in all human history to grow up with unlimited and free convenient access to high-definition porn via smartphone or tablet. In his analogy, he compared the prevalence of porn to a drug addict having a drug dealer in his pocket.

So nobody was going to come out and say that we were using porn as we sat on the balcony, but we still felt a connection to porn. It was and is still regarded as a socially acceptable unsaid vice. The barrier and potential categorization were lessened because we all knew we weren't the only ones who watched porn. Porn was difficult for me to do away with. Nobody needed to tell me it was wrong and the fact that society doesn't criminalize it (except for public usage) doesn't make it right. Any action humans act to do will often time than not be bad. I realized I didn't want to deal with issues in my life again. Porn and masturbation made things easy to gloss over. I do wonder why an addict wouldn't just stop when it becomes clear enough that his addiction is going to kill him. It wasn't the same thing to me because porn wasn't like an addiction. I believe that is why it has permeated many homes and has made relationships more mechanical. In the real sense, the similarity between porn addiction and heroin addiction is more than will care to know. The truth that I have found for myself over the years is that it takes a little amount of time for the demon of heroin to rear its head in the public glare; for its dastard effect to manifest its physical attributes.

Benefits of Porn?

I think there are areas where the distinction between education and illiteracy is hazy. Nearby my hostel, in a neighborhood gym, we had one of these. The fortunate lads met the boys who put little effort into their studies or who took advantage of the chance before losing hope. Since we have not been taught to see through a system, there is no judgment in this area. Our less fortunate brothers were not exposed to the same system that molded us as schoolboys. Truth and hypocrisy thus coexist in this place without condemnation. Why do the lads who were defrauded of a formal education speak without restraint and constantly tout the advantages of porn and masturbation. Then we accede and joined them to list the numerous benefits of our secret vices.

The association of porn with criminality, so to speak, is one advantage of porn that deserves attention.

Data showed that criminality decreases when porn is

brought into a society that would otherwise be prone to it. This demonstrates the allure of pornographic addiction. This is a macro benefit, though. Pornography is less valuable than it is harmful. Porn usage offers no benefits to the individual.

As I watch porn, the minutes turn into hours, and before long, I was spending four hours searching through various porn websites. On occasion, I had up to four website tabs open on my laptop, each specializing in horrific scenes that caught my attention.

Whenever I consume porn, I might feel elated for a while, then there comes the melancholy feelings, a gloom phase that usually ended in sleep. Then I figured it become my go to sleep stimulant. I was only deceiving myself. The REM sleep considered to be the proper type of sleep is usually unachievable after masturbation and porn usage.

Media and Porn

Perhaps the climate for porn to take hold in my life was created by my previous exposure to movies and music videos. I recalled that the majority of the films contained graphic sexual content. Around that time, the songs by Sisquo were out, oh boy! Do I hear sexual content on television? The globe was taken by the realization of the sex demand. The majority of advertising was sexual. It was as though you couldn't sell without having sex. Someone must have used sexual appeal in coffin advertisements if one searched hard enough.

Who dare underestimate the power of media? Going by the evolutionary theory understanding, manufacturers have turned things around and have based marketing on the base instincts of man. They develop innovating ways of advertising through sex. Products will either carry half-naked men or women these days.

The time we live in now is a precarious one. Tik tok, instagram, twitter, face book and so many social media platform have become mediums for soft and hard porn. All you need are keywords.

It may appear harmless to interact with sexually explicit

information on social media. It's not, I assure you. It develops a reserve of interest in you that, depending on the surrounding circumstances, might be quickly triggered. Sometimes, after watching an erotica film, I'll think I'll never again partake in masturbation or porn, but then I'll get restless and lured to the moments in the film. The scenes would frequently not be intense enough for me to experience desire and baam! I've returned to browsing pornographic websites for videos to have sex to.

The brain absorbs everything like a sponge. We must therefore be cautious about the contents we expose ourselves to. Teens consume a lot of porn, so it makes sense. This generation is especially impressionable.

Relationship and Porn

Relationships are seldom the result of one man. Relationships are essential to the existence of humans. For us to reproduce, live, and survive, we need it. No one can sustain himself alone. Silas Marner may have tried, but ultimately the destitute girl overcame his dislike of humanity. It is an uncontrollable social reality. Bonding with a real-life partner is challenging when we establish relationships with pornographic characters. We want to apply the degraded sex behaviors we observe in porn scenes to a genuine relationship. This might be quite troublesome.

These cause relationships to break up. Only when both parties are emotionally and physically invested in the relationship in a healthy way can a relationship flourish. One major element is porn.

How to Stop

You just have to stop watching porn. This will help you get your dopamine level to the baseline again. You will agree with me that you have made porn an outlet to many concerning issues in your life. You use it when you are stressed, sad and even too happy.

That's the problem, porn creeps into every part of your life hold masturbation by hand along. To stop deprive yourself of it. It might look hard. Look at it this way; deprivation is how to build a warrior mindset. Take it as a challenge to yourself and see how strong you are. You will fail, but get up and vow not to fall like a weakling again.

Deal with past trauma. It has been established that masturbation can anchor itself on some unresolved issues. It is not strange to find a rape victim with porn and masturbation problem. A depressed person can develop habit of watching porn and masturbation to hang on to life. Don't put the cart before the horse. Deal with the trauma first and it will be much more easier to resolve your porn problem.

Always be conscious of your thought. When you are

feeling bored, find something to do. Go out, take a walk, watch an interesting movie, go to the gym, take a cold shower. Do whatever it takes to get your mind off porn.